CELIAC DISEASE COOKBOOK

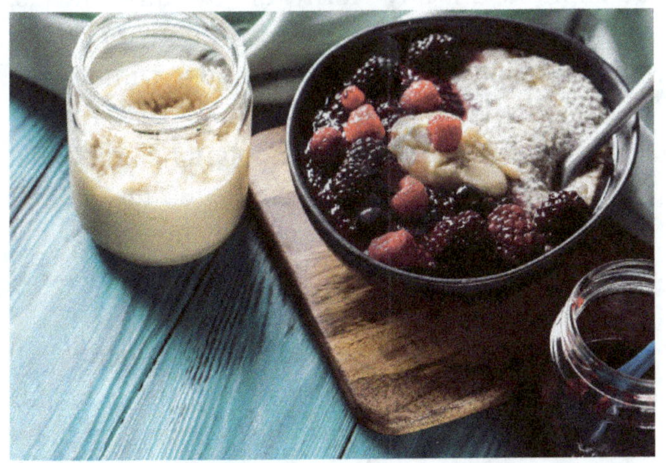

The Ultimate Guide To A Gluten-Free Lifestyle Boosting Health With Delicious Recipes And Practical Tips

Dr. Jaclyn N. Anderson

TABLE OF CONTENTS

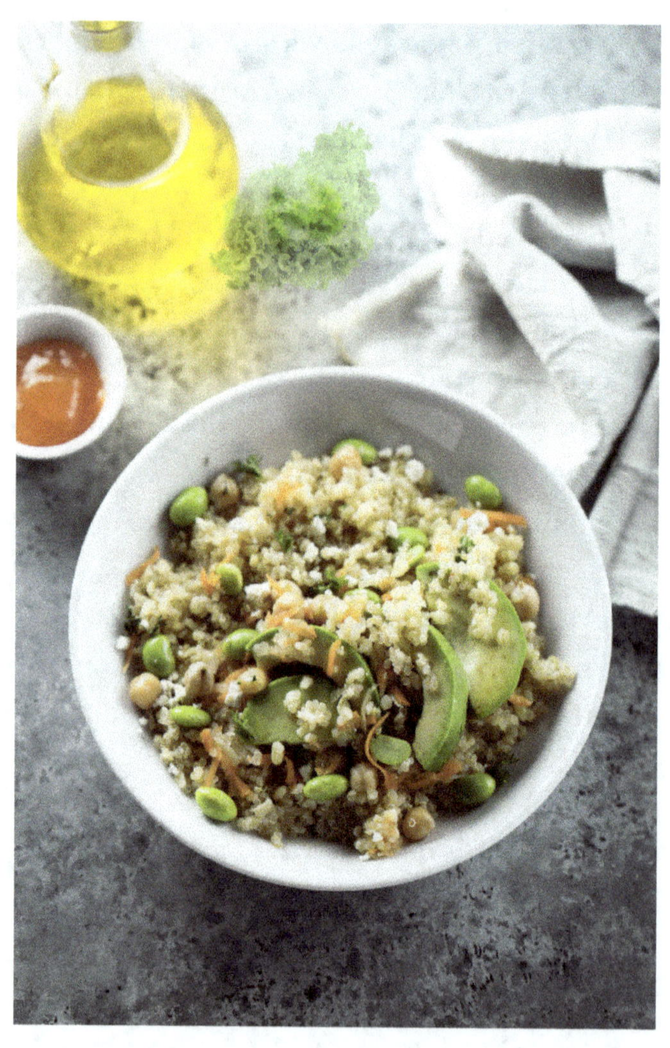

INTRODUCTION

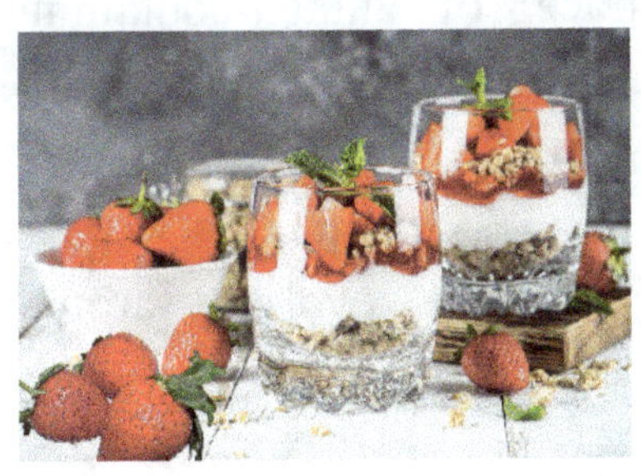

Celiac disease is an autoimmune disorder triggered by the consumption of gluten, a protein commonly found in wheat, barley, and rye. When individuals with celiac disease ingest gluten, their immune system reacts by damaging the lining of the small intestine. This damage hampers the absorption of nutrients from food, leading to various digestive issues and potential long-term health complications.

The cornerstone of managing celiac disease is adopting a strict gluten-free diet. The primary goal is to eliminate all sources of gluten from the diet to prevent intestinal damage and alleviate symptoms. This entails being vigilant about food choices and scrutinizing ingredient labels for any trace of gluten-containing substances.

The celiac disease diet revolves around naturally gluten-free foods such as fruits, vegetables, legumes, nuts, seeds, dairy products, and unprocessed meats or fish. Additionally, there is a wide array of gluten-free grains and starches available, including rice, quinoa, corn, tapioca, and gluten-free oats, which can offer diversity and necessary nutrients in the diet.

However, maintaining a gluten-free diet requires meticulous attention and awareness as gluten can often be present in unexpected products like sauces, seasonings, and processed foods. Cross-contamination during food preparation is another critical consideration as even tiny amounts of gluten can trigger adverse reactions in individuals with celiac disease.

Moreover, due to the potential nutritional deficiencies caused by malabsorption in the intestines, it's essential for those with celiac disease to work with healthcare professionals, such as dietitians or nutritionists, to ensure they receive adequate nutrients through supplements or fortified foods.

Successfully managing celiac disease through diet involves not only avoiding gluten-containing foods but also making informed, conscious dietary choices to maintain good health and overall well-being.

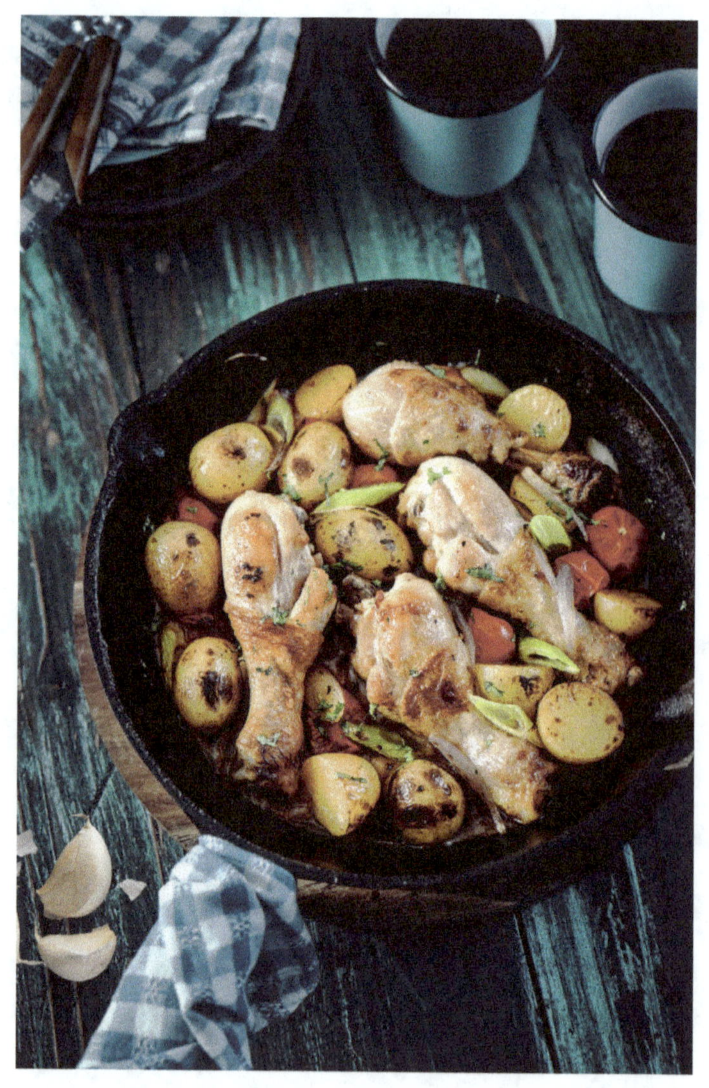

CHAPTER 1:

UNDERSTANDING CELIAC DISEASE

What is Celiac Disease?

Celiac disease is a chronic autoimmune disorder that affects the small intestine. When individuals with celiac disease consume gluten—a protein found in wheat, barley, and rye—their immune system responds by damaging the lining of the small intestine. This reaction hampers the absorption of nutrients from food.

The small finger-like projections in the small intestine, called villi, become inflamed and flattened in people with celiac disease. As a result, the surface area available for nutrient absorption decreases, leading to potential deficiencies in essential vitamins and minerals.

Causes of Celiac Disease:

Celiac disease is primarily caused by an abnormal immune system response to gluten, a protein found in wheat, barley, and rye. When individuals with a genetic predisposition to the condition consume gluten, their immune system reacts by attacking the lining of the small intestine. This response damages the tiny finger-like protrusions called villi that line the intestine. As a result, the intestine's ability to absorb nutrients is impaired.

Several factors contribute to the development of celiac disease, including genetic predisposition and environmental triggers. Having specific genes (like HLA-DQ2 and HLA-DQ8) increases the likelihood of developing the condition. However, not everyone with these genes develops celiac disease, suggesting that other environmental factors, such as certain infections or early exposure to gluten, might also play a role.

Symptoms of Celiac Disease:

Symptoms of celiac disease can vary widely among individuals, and they can manifest differently in children and adults. Some common symptoms include:

1. **Digestive problems:** This can include diarrhea, constipation, abdominal pain, bloating, gas, and nausea.

2. **Weight changes:** Unexplained weight loss or difficulty gaining weight might be observed.

3. **Fatigue and weakness:** Malabsorption of nutrients can lead to fatigue and overall weakness.

4. **Anemia:** Iron deficiency caused by poor absorption of iron from food.

5. **Skin issues:** Dermatitis herpetiformis, a chronic skin rash characterized by itchy, blistering skin.

6. Joint pain and discomfort.

7. Delayed growth and development in children.

8. **Neurological symptoms:** Some individuals may experience tingling or numbness in their hands or feet.

9. Infertility and miscarriages in women.

Diagnosis and Treatment

Diagnosis of Celiac Disease:

Diagnosing celiac disease involves several steps. Healthcare providers typically start with a thorough assessment of medical history and symptoms. If celiac disease is suspected, the following diagnostic steps are commonly taken:

1. **Blood Tests:** A blood test screens for specific antibodies that the body produces in response to gluten. Elevated levels of these antibodies, such as tissue transglutaminase (tTG) and deamidated gliadin peptide (DGP) antibodies, can indicate an immune response to gluten.

2. **Genetic Testing:** Testing for the presence of the HLA-DQ2 and HLA-DQ8 genes, which are strongly associated with celiac disease, might be done. However, having these genes doesn't necessarily mean a person will develop celiac disease.

3. **Intestinal Biopsy:** If blood tests suggest celiac disease, a gastroenterologist might perform an endoscopy to take small samples (biopsies) of the small intestine's lining. This is the most definitive test for diagnosing celiac disease. The biopsies

help evaluate the damage to the villi and confirm the diagnosis.

Treatment of Celiac Disease:

The only effective treatment for celiac disease is a strict gluten-free diet. This involves completely avoiding foods and products containing wheat, barley, and rye. Even small amounts of gluten can trigger an immune response and worsen intestinal damage.

A gluten-free diet allows the small intestine to heal and reduces symptoms. It's crucial for those with celiac disease to be diligent in checking food labels and ensuring that the food they consume is gluten-free. This diet often involves consuming naturally gluten-free foods such as fruits, vegetables, meats, fish, poultry, dairy, and gluten-free grains like rice or quinoa.

In some cases, individuals might also need to supplement their diet with vitamins and minerals, particularly if deficiencies exist due to malabsorption. Regular follow-ups with healthcare providers, such as dietitians and gastroenterologists, are recommended to monitor the condition and ensure nutritional needs are met.

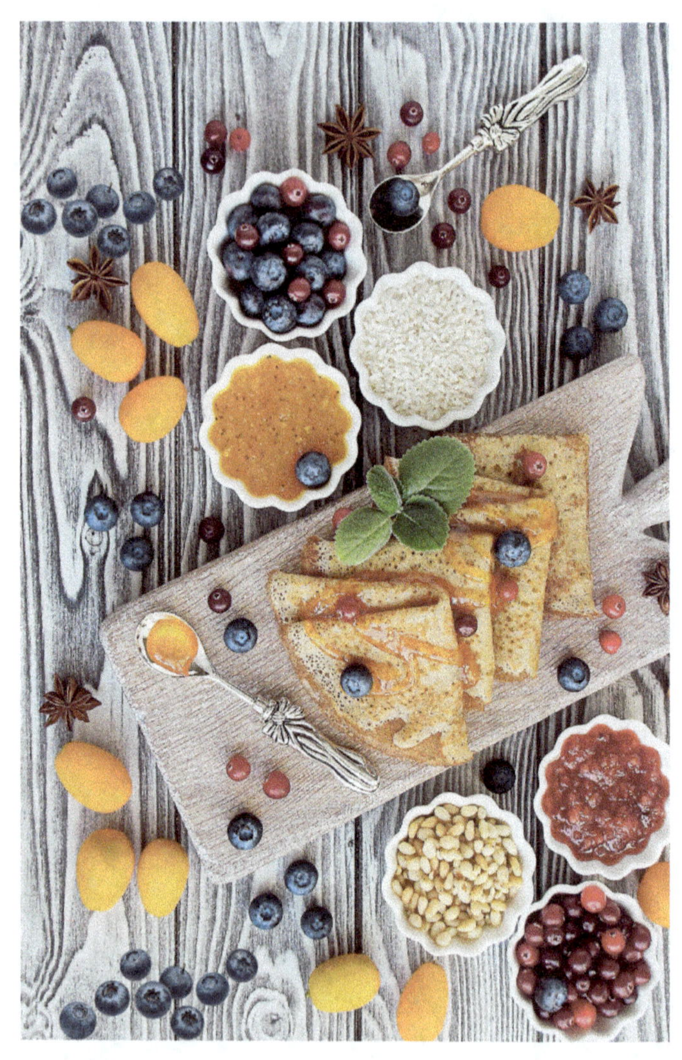

CHAPTER 2:

SETTING UP A GLUTEN-FREE KITCHEN

Stocking Your Pantry

Gluten-Free Flours:

1. **Rice Flour:** Both white and brown rice flour are versatile and commonly used in gluten-free baking.

2. **Almond Flour:** Adds moisture and richness to baked goods.

3. **Coconut Flour:** Absorbs moisture and adds flavor.

4. **Tapioca Flour/Starch:** Enhances texture and structure in baking.

5. **Corn Flour or Cornmeal:** Used in various dishes like cornbread and as a coating for frying.

Whole Grains:

1. **Quinoa:** A protein-rich and versatile grain used in salads, pilafs, or as a side dish.

2. **Millet:** Nutritious and gluten-free grain suitable for porridge or in baking.

3. **Buckwheat:** Despite its name, it's gluten-free and great for pancakes, noodles, or as a side dish.

Starches and Thickeners:

1. **Potato Starch:** Adds lightness to baked goods and is used as a thickening agent.

2. **Arrowroot Powder:** Serves as a thickener for sauces, gravies, and puddings.

Gluten-Free Pasta and Noodles:

1. Look for various options made from rice, corn, quinoa, or legumes.

Proteins:

1. **Beans and Lentils:** Versatile and nutrient-rich for soups, salads, or main dishes.

2. **Meat, Poultry, and Fish:** Naturally gluten-free protein sources.

Dairy and Dairy Alternatives:

1. **Milk, Yogurt, and Cheese:** Most dairy products are naturally gluten-free.

2. **Plant-Based Milk (Almond, Coconut, Soy):** Check for gluten-free labeling.

Healthy Fats and Oils:

1. **Olive Oil, Avocado Oil, and Coconut Oil:** Versatile for cooking and dressing.

2. **Butter and Ghee:** Check for cross-contamination if extreme sensitivity exists.

Flavor Enhancers:

1. **Herbs and Spices:** Fresh or dried, for adding flavor to dishes.
2. **Gluten-Free Soy Sauce or Tamari:** Essential for seasoning and marinades.

Sweeteners:

1. **Sugar, Honey, Maple Syrup:** Pure forms without additives are typically gluten-free.
2. **Stevia, Agave, or Molasses:** Alternative sweeteners to explore.

Baking Essentials:

1. **Baking Powder, Baking Soda:** Check for gluten-free certification.
2. **Vanilla Extract, Cocoa Powder:** For adding flavor to baked goods.

List Of Foods To Avoid

1. **Wheat-Based Products:** Wheat in all forms, including bread, flour, pasta, couscous, and wheat-based cereals.

2. **Barley and Rye Products:** Barley, such as malt, malt vinegar, malt extract, and some beer. Rye in bread, crackers, and cereals.

3. **Processed Foods with Hidden Gluten:** Many processed and packaged foods might contain hidden gluten, such as sauces, soups, salad dressings, and processed meats like sausages and hot dogs.

4. **Baked Goods and Pastries:** Cakes, cookies, pastries, pies, and certain desserts made with regular flour.

5. **Some Grains and Flours:** Spelt, semolina, einkorn, and farro are varieties of wheat and contain gluten.

6. **Regular flour:** unless labeled specifically as gluten-free.

7. **Breaded or Coated Foods:** Foods that are breaded or coated, like fried chicken or fish, often contain gluten.

8. **Certain Beverages:** Regular beer, some malted beverages, and certain mixed drinks containing alcohol made from gluten grains.

9. Some non-dairy milk substitutes might contain gluten, so check labels.

10. **Processed Snack Foods:** Some snacks like pretzels, crackers, and certain flavored chips might contain gluten.

11. **Sauces and Condiments:** Soy sauce, unless specifically labeled as gluten-free tamari or a wheat-free alternative.

12. Some salad dressings and gravies may contain gluten.

13. **Deli Meats and Processed Meats:** Some deli meats and sausages might have added fillers that contain gluten.

Kitchen Equipment and Utensils

1. **Dedicated Kitchen Tools:** Have separate cutting boards, toasters, and cooking utensils specifically designated for gluten-free use. Color-coding or clearly marking these items can help differentiate them from those used for gluten-containing foods.

2. **Cookware and Bakeware:** Consider having separate pots, pans, baking sheets, and muffin tins for gluten-free cooking. Stainless steel or cast iron cookware that can be thoroughly cleaned might be ideal.

3. **Colanders and Strainers:** Have separate colanders for draining gluten-

free pasta, vegetables, or grains to avoid cross-contact with gluten residues.

4. **Toaster and Toaster Bags:** Consider using a dedicated gluten-free toaster or toaster bags to prevent cross-contamination when toasting bread or other items.

5. **Mixing Bowls and Food Processors:** Use separate mixing bowls, food processors, and blenders for preparing gluten-free meals.

6. **Storage Containers and Labels:** Store gluten-free ingredients in clearly labeled containers to prevent mix-ups and cross-contamination.

7. **Cleaning Supplies:** Have separate sponges, dishcloths, and towels for cleaning surfaces used in gluten-free food preparation.

8. **Labeling and Organization:** Keep gluten-free items well-organized and

clearly labeled in the pantry and refrigerator to avoid confusion or accidental use of gluten-containing products.

9. **Kitchen Hygiene:** Practice regular and thorough cleaning of all kitchen surfaces, including countertops, stove-tops, and utensil drawers, to eliminate any gluten residues.

10. **Education and Communication:** Ensure that everyone who uses the kitchen is aware of the importance of maintaining a gluten-free environment and the risks associated with cross-contamination.

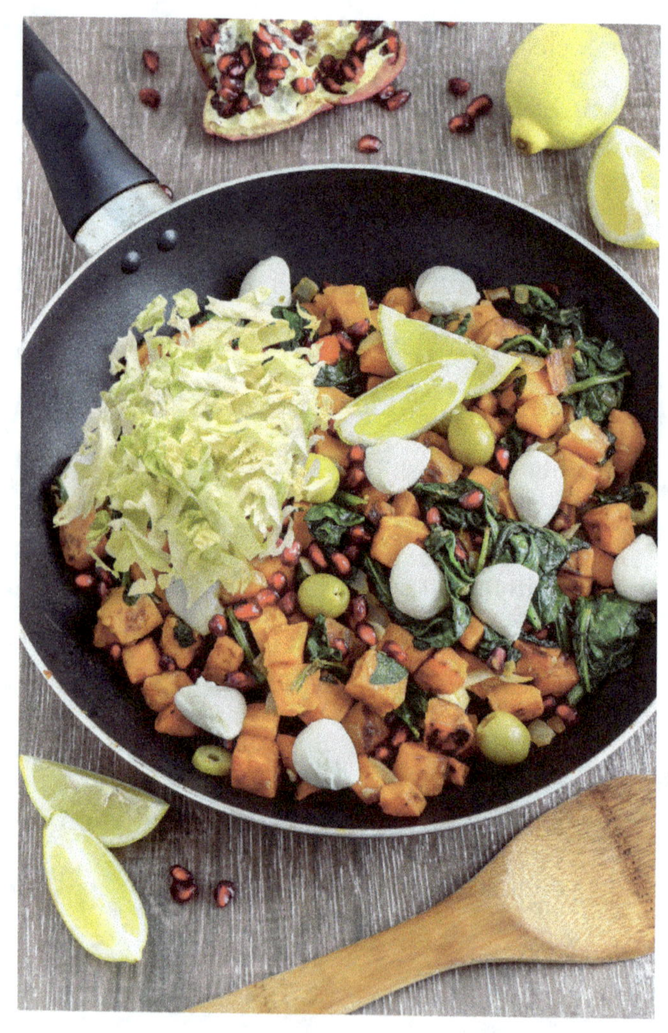

CHAPTER 3:

BREAKFAST DELIGHTS

Quinoa Breakfast Bowl

Ingredients:

- 1 cup quinoa
- 2 cups almond milk
- 2 tablespoons honey
- 1 teaspoon cinnamon
- Fresh fruits (berries, banana slices)
- Nuts (almonds, walnuts)
- Chia seeds

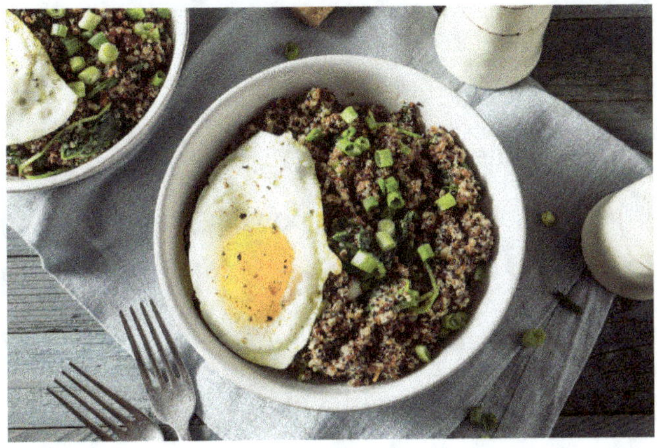

Nutritional Information (per serving):

Calories	Protein	Carbs	Fat	Fiber
320	8g	52g	9g	6g

Preparation:

1. Rinse the quinoa and cook it in almond milk according to package instructions.
2. Stir in honey and cinnamon.
3. Serve in bowls, topped with fruits, nuts, and a sprinkle of chia seeds.

Gluten-Free Pancakes

Ingredients:

- 1 cup gluten-free flour
- 1 tablespoon sugar
- 1 teaspoon baking powder
- 1 egg
- 1 cup almond milk
- 1 teaspoon vanilla extract
- Berries or sliced bananas (optional)

Nutritional Information (per serving):

Calories	Protein	Carbs	Fat	Fiber
180	4g	30g	5g	2g

Preparation:

1. Mix flour, sugar, and baking powder in a bowl.

2. Add egg, almond milk, and vanilla extract, whisk until smooth.

3. Heat a non-stick pan, pour batter, cook until bubbles form, flip and cook until golden.

4. Serve with fresh fruits if desired.

Egg Muffins

Ingredients:

- 6 eggs
- 1/4 cup chopped spinach
- 1/4 cup diced bell peppers

- 1/4 cup diced ham or cooked sausage
- Salt and pepper to taste

Nutritional Information (per serving, 2 muffins):

Calories	Protein	Carbs	Fat	Fiber
150	12g	3g	9g	1g

Preparation:

1. Preheat the oven to 350°F (175°C). Grease a muffin tin.
2. Whisk eggs, mix in veggies, meat, salt, and pepper.
3. Pour the mixture into the muffin cups.
4. Bake for 20-25 minutes or until the muffins are set.
5. Let them cool slightly before removing from the tin.

Chia Seed Pudding

Ingredients:

- 1/4 cup chia seeds
- 1 cup almond milk
- 1 tablespoon honey or maple syrup
- 1/2 teaspoon vanilla extract
- Sliced fruits or nuts for topping

Nutritional Information (per serving):

Calories	Protein	Carbs	Fat	Fiber
210	6g	25g	10g	12g

Preparation:

1. Mix chia seeds, almond milk, sweetener, and vanilla in a jar.
2. Stir well, cover, and refrigerate for at least 2 hours or overnight.
3. Top with fruits or nuts before serving.

Greek Yogurt Parfait

Ingredients:

- 1 cup Greek yogurt
- 1/4 cup gluten-free granola
- 1/2 cup mixed berries
- Honey (optional)

Nutritional Information (per serving):

Calories	Protein	Carbs	Fat	Fiber
250	18g	30g	8g	4g

Preparation:

1. Layer yogurt, granola, and berries in a glass or bowl.
2. Drizzle honey if desired.
3. Repeat the layers and serve chilled.

Sweet Potato Hash

Ingredients:

- 2 medium sweet potatoes, peeled and diced
- 1 bell pepper, diced
- 1 onion, chopped
- 2 tablespoons olive oil
- 1 teaspoon paprika
- Salt and pepper to taste
- Fresh parsley for garnish

Nutritional Information (per serving):

Calories	Protein	Carbs	Fat	Fiber
220	3g	35g	8g	5g

Preparation:

1. Heat olive oil in a skillet over medium heat.
2. Add sweet potatoes, bell pepper, and onion. Cook until the sweet potatoes are tender.
3. Season with paprika, salt, and pepper.

4. Garnish with fresh parsley before serving.

Avocado Toast

Ingredients:

- 2 slices gluten-free bread
- 1 ripe avocado
- Lemon juice
- Red pepper flakes (optional)
- Salt and pepper to taste

Nutritional Information (per serving):

Calories	Protein	Carbs	Fat	Fiber
280	5g	25g	18g	8g

Preparation:

1. Toast the gluten-free bread.
2. Mash the avocado with a fork, add lemon juice, salt, and pepper.
3. Spread the avocado mixture on the toast.

4. Sprinkle with red pepper flakes if desired.

Rice Cake with Almond Butter and Berries

Ingredients:

- 2 rice cakes
- 2 tablespoons almond butter
- Mixed berries
- Honey (optional)

Nutritional Information (per serving):

Calories	Protein	Carbs	Fat	Fiber
240	6g	30g	11g	5g

Preparation:

1. Spread almond butter evenly on the rice cakes.
2. Top with mixed berries.
3. Drizzle with honey for added sweetness.

Egg and Veggie Breakfast Wraps

Ingredients:

- 4 gluten-free wraps
- 4 eggs, scrambled
- 1 cup sautéed mixed vegetables (bell peppers, spinach, mushrooms)
- Salsa (optional)
- Avocado slices (optional)

Nutritional Information (per serving):

Calories	Protein	Carbs	Fat	Fiber
310	12g	30g	15g	6g

Preparation:

1. Lay out the wraps, add scrambled eggs and mixed veggies.
2. Add salsa and avocado if desired.
3. Roll up the wraps and serve.

Coconut Flour Waffles

Ingredients:

- 1 cup coconut flour
- 1 teaspoon baking powder
- 4 eggs
- 1 cup almond milk
- 2 tablespoons honey or maple syrup
- Berries for topping

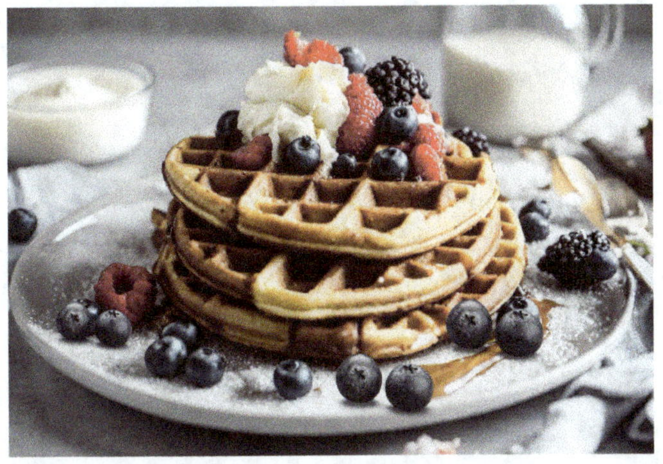

Nutritional Information (per serving):

Calories	Protein	Carbs	Fat	Fiber
260	12g	30g	10g	8g

Preparation:

1. Mix coconut flour and baking powder.

2. Add eggs, almond milk, and sweetener. Combine until smooth.

3. Cook in a preheated waffle iron according to the manufacturer's instructions.

4. Top with fresh berries before serving.

Buckwheat Porridge

Ingredients:

- 1/2 cup buckwheat groats
- 1 cup water or milk of choice
- 1 tablespoon honey or maple syrup
- Sliced fruits (apples, berries)
- Cinnamon (optional)

Nutritional Information (per serving):

Calories	Protein	Carbs	Fat	Fiber
220	6g	45g	2g	6g

Preparation:

1. Rinse buckwheat and combine it with water or milk in a pot. Bring to a boil, then simmer for 15-20 minutes until tender.
2. Sweeten with honey or maple syrup.
3. Top with sliced fruits and a sprinkle of cinnamon.

Omelet with Spinach and Feta

Ingredients:

- 3 eggs
- Handful of fresh spinach
- 2 tablespoons crumbled feta cheese
- Salt and pepper to taste
- Fresh herbs (parsley or dill) for garnish

Nutritional Information (per serving):

Calories	Protein	Carbs	Fat	Fiber

270	18g	3g	20g	1g

Preparation:

1. Beat the eggs and season with salt and pepper.

2. Heat a pan, add spinach and cook until wilted.

3. Pour in the eggs and sprinkle feta over the top.

4. Cook until the omelet sets, then fold it in half.

5. Garnish with fresh herbs before serving.

Smoothie Bowl

Ingredients:

- 1 frozen banana
- 1/2 cup mixed berries
- 1/2 cup almond milk
- Toppings: sliced fruits, nuts, shredded coconut

Nutritional Information (approximate, without toppings):

Calories	Protein	Carbs	Fat	Fiber
200	3g	45g	3g	8g

Preparation:

1. Blend the frozen banana, berries, and almond milk until smooth.
2. Pour the smoothie into a bowl.
3. Top with sliced fruits, nuts, and shredded coconut.

Breakfast Quinoa Muffins

Ingredients:

- 1 cup cooked quinoa
- 2 eggs
- 1/2 cup spinach, chopped
- 1/4 cup shredded cheese
- Salt and pepper to taste

Nutritional Information (per serving, 2 muffins):

Calories	Protein	Carbs	Fat	Fiber
180	12g	15g	8g	2g

Preparation:

1. Preheat oven to 350°F (175°C). Grease a muffin tin.
2. In a bowl, mix quinoa, eggs, spinach, cheese, salt, and pepper.
3. Spoon the mixture into the muffin cups.
4. Bake for 20-25 minutes or until set.

Sautéed Banana Slices with Cinnamon

Ingredients:

- 2 ripe bananas, sliced
- 1 tablespoon coconut oil
- 1 teaspoon cinnamon

- Optional toppings: Greek yogurt, nuts, honey

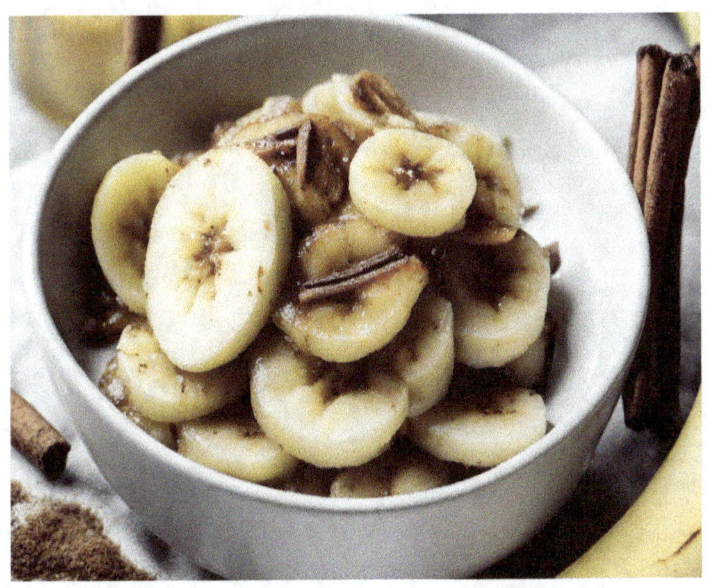

Nutritional Information (per serving):

Calories	Protein	Carbs	Fat	Fiber
180	2g	30g	7g	4g

Preparation:

1. Heat coconut oil in a pan over medium heat.

2. Add banana slices and sprinkle with cinnamon.

3. Sauté until golden and slightly caramelized.

4. Serve alone or with toppings like Greek yogurt, nuts, or honey.

CHAPTER 4:

APPETIZERS AND SNACKS

Guacamole with Veggie Sticks

Ingredients:

- 3 ripe avocados

- 1 lime (juiced)

- 1/2 red onion (finely chopped)

- 2 tomatoes (deseeded and diced)

- Fresh cilantro (chopped)

- Salt and pepper to taste

- Carrot and cucumber sticks

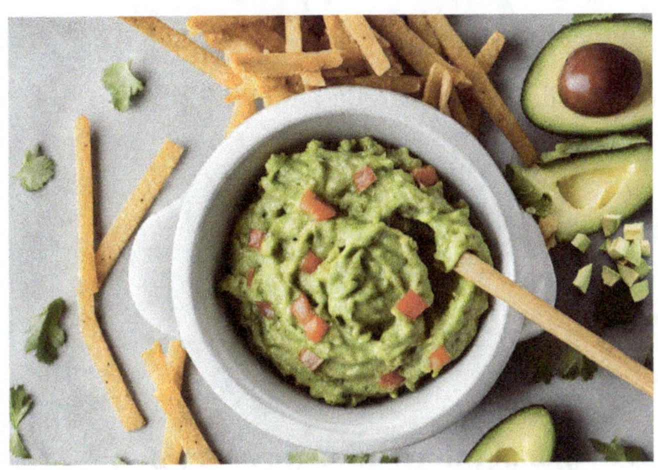

Nutritional Information (per serving): Guacamole Only:

Calories	Protein	Carbs	Fat	Fiber
120	2g	7g	10g	5g

Preparation:

1. Mash avocados with lime juice.
2. Add onion, tomatoes, cilantro, salt, and pepper. Mix well.
3. Serve with carrot and cucumber sticks.

Caprese Skewers

Ingredients:

- Fresh mozzarella balls
- Cherry tomatoes
- Fresh basil leaves
- Balsamic glaze
- Skewers

Nutritional Information (per serving):

Calories	Protein	Carbs	Fat	Fiber
150	8g	4g	10g	1g

Preparation:

1. Thread mozzarella, tomatoes, and basil onto skewers.
2. Drizzle with balsamic glaze before serving.

Stuffed Mini Peppers

Ingredients:

- Mini bell peppers
- Cream cheese (or dairy-free alternative)
- Chopped chives
- Garlic powder
- Paprika
- Salt and pepper

Nutritional Information (per serving):

Calories	Protein	Carbs	Fat	Fiber

90	2g	6g	7g	1g

Preparation:

1. Preheat oven to 375°F (190°C).

2. Cut the tops off the peppers, remove seeds, and membranes.

3. Mix cream cheese, chives, garlic powder, paprika, salt, and pepper.

4. Stuff the peppers and bake for 10-12 minutes until softened.

Deviled Eggs

Ingredients:

- Hard-boiled eggs
- Mayonnaise (or Greek yogurt)
- Dijon mustard
- Paprika
- Chopped chives (for garnish)

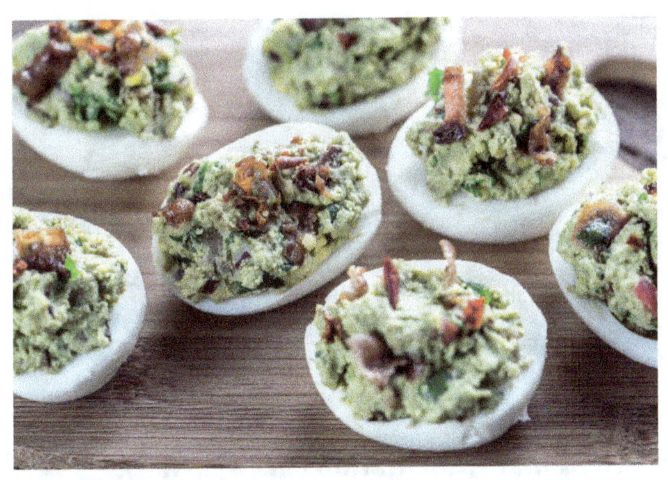

Nutritional Information (per serving, 2 halves):

Calories	Protein	Carbs	Fat	Fiber
100	6g	1g	8g	0g

Preparation:

1. Slice eggs in half, remove yolks, and mash with mayo, mustard, and a sprinkle of paprika.

2. Fill egg white halves with the yolk mixture.

3. Garnish with chives before serving.

Smoked Salmon Cucumber Bites

Ingredients:

- English cucumbers
- Smoked salmon
- Cream cheese (or dairy-free alternative)
- Dill (for garnish)

Nutritional Information (per serving):

Calories	Protein	Carbs	Fat	Fiber
80	5g	2g	6g	0g

Preparation:

1. Slice cucumbers into rounds, top each with a small amount of cream cheese.
2. Place a piece of smoked salmon on top.
3. Garnish with fresh dill.

Roasted Chickpeas

Ingredients:

- 1 can chickpeas (drained and rinsed)

- Olive oil
- Salt
- Seasonings (paprika, cumin, garlic powder)

Nutritional Information (per serving):

Calories	Protein	Carbs	Fat	Fiber
120	6g	18g	3g	5g

Preparation:

1. Preheat the oven to 400°F (200°C).
2. Dry chickpeas, toss with olive oil and seasonings.
3. Roast on a baking sheet for 25-30 minutes until crispy.

Quinoa Sushi Rolls

Ingredients:

- Nori sheets
- Cooked quinoa

- Sliced veggies (cucumber, avocado, bell pepper)
- Rice vinegar
- Gluten-free soy sauce (tamari)

Nutritional Information (per serving):

Calories	Protein	Carbs	Fat	Fiber
160	5g	25g	4g	5g

Preparation:

1. Lay out a nori sheet, spread quinoa, add veggies.
2. Roll tightly and slice into pieces.
3. Serve with a side of tamari for dipping.

Spinach and Artichoke Dip

Ingredients:

- Frozen spinach (thawed and drained)
- Canned artichoke hearts (chopped)
- Cream cheese (or dairy-free alternative)

- Mayonnaise

- Garlic powder

- Shredded cheese (optional)

Nutritional Information (per serving):

Calories	Protein	Carbs	Fat	Fiber
140	4g	6g	10g	2g

Preparation:

1. Mix spinach, artichokes, cream cheese, mayo, and garlic powder in a baking dish.

2. Top with shredded cheese if desired and bake at 350°F (175°C) until bubbly.

Baked Zucchini Chips

Ingredients:

- Zucchini, thinly sliced

- Olive oil

- Gluten-free breadcrumbs

- Garlic powder

- Parmesan cheese (or nutritional yeast for dairy-free)

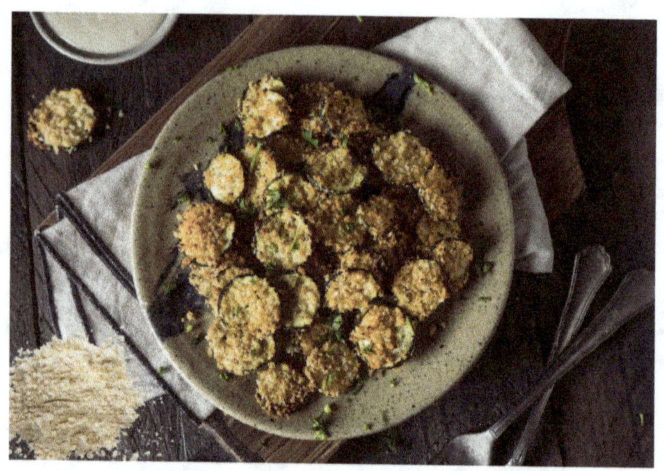

Nutritional Information (per serving):

Calories	Protein	Carbs	Fat	Fiber
90	3g	8g	5g	2g

Preparation:

1. Preheat oven to 425°F (220°C).

2. Toss zucchini slices in olive oil, then coat with breadcrumbs, garlic powder, and parmesan.

3. Bake on a baking sheet until golden and
   crisp.

Hummus with Gluten-Free Crackers

Ingredients:

- Store-bought or homemade hummus
- Gluten-free crackers
- Optional: Drizzle of olive oil, paprika, or
  pine nuts for garnish

Nutritional Information (per serving):

Calories	Protein	Carbs	Fat	Fiber
160	4g	20g	8g	4g

Preparation:

1. Arrange hummus in a bowl, drizzle with
   olive oil and sprinkle with paprika or
   pine nuts if desired.
2. Serve with gluten-free crackers for
   dipping.

Crispy Kale Chips

Ingredients:

- Fresh kale, stems removed and torn into pieces
- Olive oil
- Salt
- Optional: Garlic powder, nutritional yeast

Nutritional Information (per serving):

Calories	Protein	Carbs	Fat	Fiber
60	3g	7g	3g	2g

Preparation:

1. Preheat the oven to 275°F (135°C).
2. Massage kale with olive oil and spread on a baking sheet.
3. Sprinkle it with salt and optional seasonings.
4. Bake for 20-25 minutes until crispy.

Fruit Skewers with Yogurt Dip

Ingredients:

- Assorted fruits (strawberries, pineapple, grapes, etc.)
- Wooden skewers
- Greek yogurt (or dairy-free yogurt)
- Honey (optional for sweetening)

Nutritional Information (per serving):

Calories	Protein	Carbs	Fat	Fiber
120	3g	25g	1g	3g

Preparation:

1. Thread mixed fruits onto skewers.
2. Mix yogurt with honey if desired and serve as a dip for the fruit skewers.

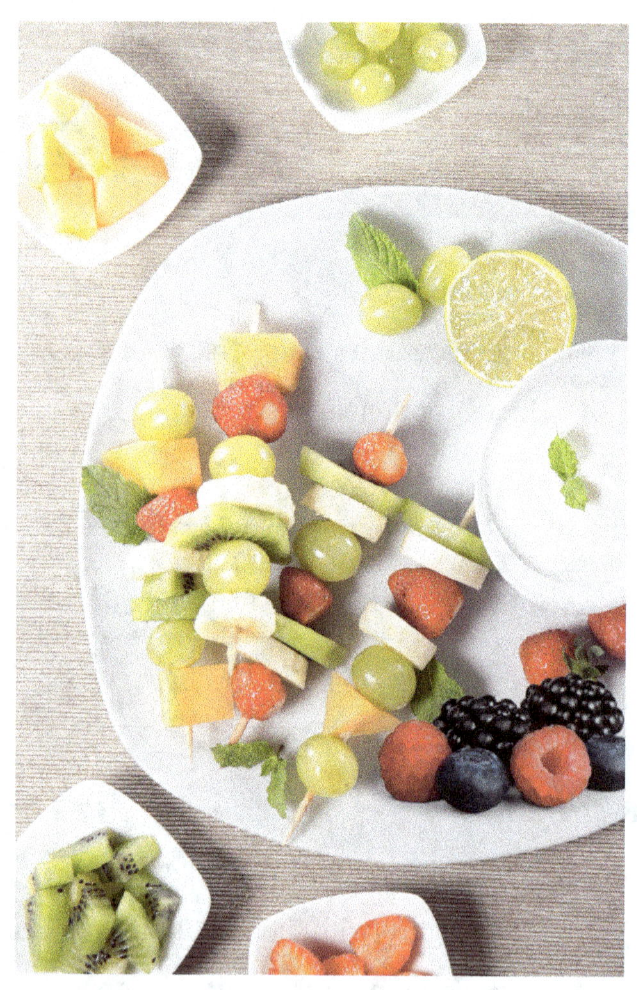

CHAPTER 5:

SATISFYING SOUPS AND SALADS

Soups:

Gluten-Free Chicken and Vegetable Soup

Ingredients:

- 1 pound boneless, skinless chicken breasts
- 8 cups gluten-free chicken broth
- 2 carrots, diced
- 2 celery stalks, diced
- 1 onion, diced
- 2 cloves garlic, minced
- 1 teaspoon dried thyme
- Salt and pepper to taste
- Fresh parsley for garnish

Nutritional Information (per serving):

Calories	Protein	Carbs	Fat	Fiber
180	25g	6g	5g	1g

Preparation:

1. In a large pot, combine chicken, broth, carrots, celery, onion, garlic, thyme, salt, and pepper.
2. Bring to a boil, then reduce heat and simmer for 20-25 minutes until chicken is cooked.
3. Remove the chicken, shred it, and return it to the pot.
4. Serve garnished with fresh parsley.

Quinoa and Vegetable Soup

Ingredients:

- 1 cup quinoa, rinsed
- 6 cups gluten-free vegetable broth
- 2 carrots, diced
- 2 celery stalks, diced

- 1 onion, chopped
- 2 cloves garlic, minced
- 1 teaspoon cumin
- 1 teaspoon paprika
- Salt and pepper to taste
- Fresh cilantro for garnish

Nutritional Information (per serving):

Calories	Protein	Carbs	Fat	Fiber
220	6g	35g	5g	6g

Preparation:

1. In a pot, combine quinoa, broth, carrots, celery, onion, garlic, cumin, paprika, salt, and pepper.
2. Bring to a boil, then simmer for 15-20 minutes until quinoa and vegetables are tender.
3. Serve garnished with fresh cilantro.

Tomato Basil Soup

Ingredients:

- 6 large tomatoes, chopped
- 1 onion, chopped
- 3 cloves garlic, minced
- 4 cups gluten-free vegetable broth
- 1/4 cup fresh basil, chopped
- 2 tablespoons olive oil
- Salt and pepper to taste
- Optional: Coconut milk for creaminess

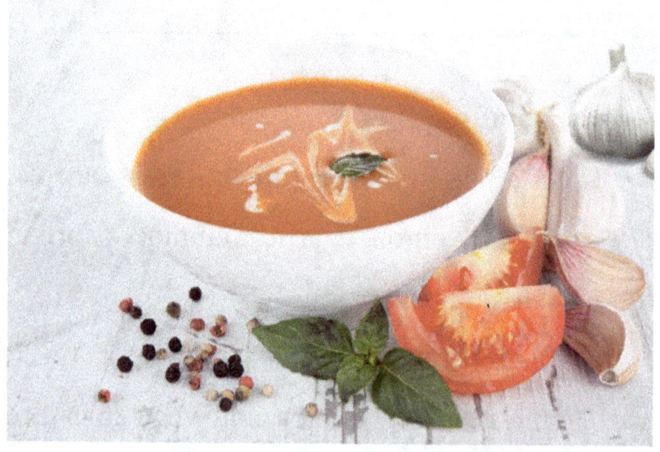

Nutritional Information (per serving):

Calories	Protein	Carbs	Fat	Fiber

120	3g	15g	6g	4g

Preparation:

1. In a pot, heat olive oil and sauté onion and garlic until soft.

2. Add tomatoes, broth, basil, salt, and pepper. Simmer for 20-25 minutes.

3. Blend until smooth. Add coconut milk if desired for creaminess before serving.

Butternut Squash Soup

Ingredients:

- 1 butternut squash, peeled and cubed
- 1 onion, chopped
- 2 carrots, chopped
- 4 cups gluten-free vegetable broth
- 1 teaspoon ground cinnamon
- 1/2 teaspoon ground nutmeg
- Olive oil
- Salt and pepper to taste

- Roasted pumpkin seeds for garnish

Nutritional Information (per serving):

Calories	Protein	Carbs	Fat	Fiber
160	2g	30g	5g	6g

Preparation:

1. Roast the squash, onion, and carrots with olive oil, salt, and pepper until tender.
2. Blend the roasted veggies with broth, cinnamon, and nutmeg until smooth.
3. Reheat the mixture in a pot, adjust seasoning, and serve garnished with roasted pumpkin seeds.

Salads:

Mediterranean Quinoa Salad

Ingredients:

- 1 cup cooked quinoa
- Cucumber, diced

- Cherry tomatoes, halved

- Red onion, thinly sliced

- Kalamata olives

- Feta cheese (optional)

- Fresh parsley, chopped

- Olive oil and lemon juice for dressing

Nutritional Information (per serving):

Calories	Protein	Carbs	Fat	Fiber
250	6g	30g	10g	5g

Preparation:

1. Combine quinoa, cucumber, tomatoes, onion, olives, and feta in a bowl.

2. Drizzle with olive oil and lemon juice, toss well.

3. Garnish with fresh parsley before serving.

Kale and Chickpea Salad

Ingredients:

- Fresh kale, stems removed and chopped
- 1 can chickpeas, drained and rinsed
- Grated carrots
- Sunflower seeds
- Dried cranberries
- Balsamic vinaigrette

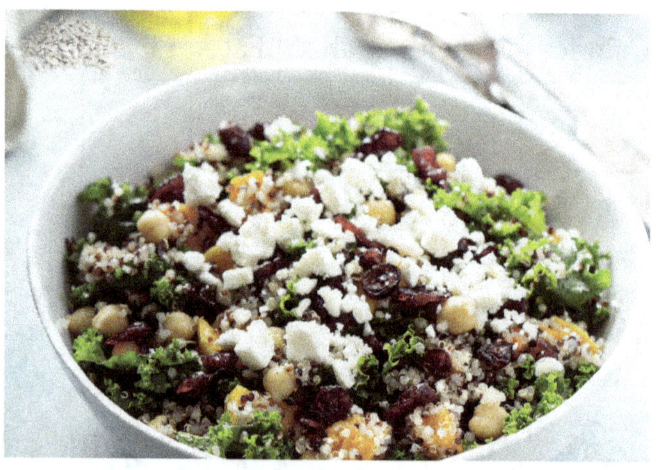

Nutritional Information (per serving):

Calories	Protein	Carbs	Fat	Fiber
220	8g	30g	8g	7g

Preparation:

1. Massage kale with a bit of olive oil to soften.
2. Toss kale with chickpeas, carrots, sunflower seeds, and cranberries.
3. Drizzle with balsamic vinaigrette before serving.

Grilled Chicken and Avocado Salad

Ingredients:

- Grilled chicken breast, sliced
- Mixed salad greens
- Cherry tomatoes, halved
- Avocado, sliced
- Red bell pepper, sliced
- Cucumber, sliced
- Balsamic dressing

Nutritional Information (per serving):

Calories	Protein	Carbs	Fat	Fiber

280	25g	15g	15g	8g

Preparation:

1. Arrange salad greens on a plate, top with grilled chicken, tomatoes, avocado, bell pepper, and cucumber.

2. Drizzle with balsamic dressing before serving.

Tuna and White Bean Salad

Ingredients:

- Canned white beans, drained and rinsed
- Canned tuna, drained
- Red onion, finely chopped
- Chopped parsley
- Lemon juice
- Olive oil
- Salt and pepper to taste

Nutritional Information (per serving):

Calories	Protein	Carbs	Fat	Fiber
230	25g	20g	8g	6g

Preparation:

1. Combine white beans, tuna, onion, and parsley in a bowl.
2. Drizzle with lemon juice and olive oil, season with salt and pepper.
3. Toss gently and serve.

Greek Salad

Ingredients:

- Cucumber, diced
- Cherry tomatoes, halved
- Red onion, thinly sliced
- Kalamata olives
- Feta cheese
- Fresh oregano
- Olive oil and red wine vinegar for dressing

Nutritional Information (per serving):

Calories	Protein	Carbs	Fat	Fiber
180	6g	10g	12g	3g

Preparation:

1. Combine cucumber, tomatoes, onion, olives, and feta in a bowl.
2. Sprinkle with fresh oregano, dress with olive oil and vinegar, toss well before serving.

Asian Noodle Salad

Ingredients:

- Gluten-free noodles (rice or soba)
- Shredded cabbage
- Shredded carrots
- Edamame
- Sliced green onions
- Sesame seeds

- Soy sauce or tamari

- Rice vinegar

- Sesame oil

Nutritional Information (per serving):

Calories	Protein	Carbs	Fat	Fiber
280	10g	35g	10g	6g

Preparation:

1. Cook noodles according to package instructions, then rinse and drain.

2. Combine noodles, cabbage, carrots, edamame, and green onions in a bowl.

3. Make a dressing with soy sauce, rice vinegar, and sesame oil. Toss the salad with the dressing and sprinkle sesame seeds before serving.

Spinach and Strawberry Salad

Ingredients:

- Fresh spinach leaves

- Sliced strawberries

- Sliced almonds

- Feta cheese (optional)

- Balsamic vinaigrette

Nutritional Information (per serving):

Calories	Protein	Carbs	Fat	Fiber
150	5g	12g	9g	4g

Preparation:

1. Arrange spinach on a plate, top with sliced strawberries, almonds, and feta.
2. Drizzle with balsamic vinaigrette before serving.

Cobb Salad

Ingredients:

- Mixed salad greens

- Grilled chicken, diced

- Hard-boiled eggs, chopped

- Avocado, diced

- Cherry tomatoes, halved

- Cooked bacon, crumbled

- Blue cheese (or dairy-free alternative), crumbled

- Ranch dressing

Nutritional Information (per serving):

Calories	Protein	Carbs	Fat	Fiber
320	25g	10g	20g	6g

Preparation:

1. Arrange salad greens on a plate, then top with rows of chicken, eggs, avocado, tomatoes, bacon, and blue cheese.
2. Drizzle with ranch dressing before serving.

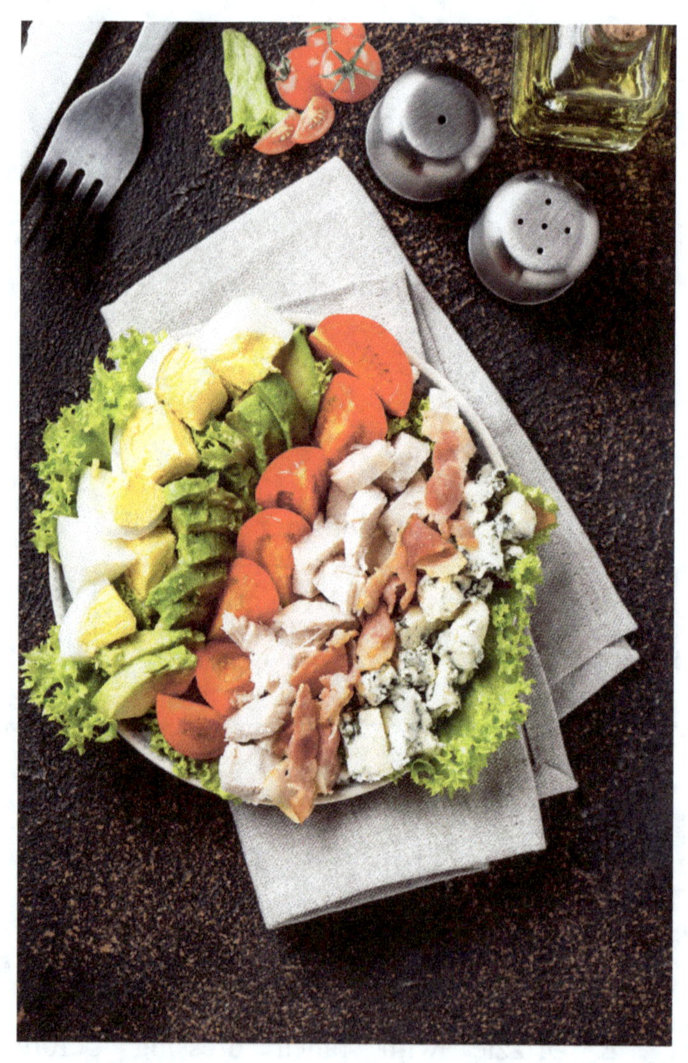

CHAPTER 6:

MAIN COURSES

Wholesome Grains and Pasta

Quinoa Stuffed Bell Peppers

Ingredients:

- 4 bell peppers, tops removed and seeds removed
- 1 cup quinoa, rinsed
- 2 cups gluten-free vegetable broth
- 1 can black beans, drained and rinsed
- 1 cup corn kernels
- 1 can diced tomatoes
- 1 teaspoon cumin
- 1 teaspoon chili powder
- Salt and pepper to taste
- Shredded cheese (optional)

Nutritional Information (per serving, 1 stuffed pepper):

Calories	Protein	Carbs	Fat	Fiber
280	10g	50g	4g	10g

Preparation:

1. Preheat the oven to 375°F (190°C).

2. In a pot, combine quinoa and broth, bring to a boil, then simmer for 15-20 minutes until liquid is absorbed.

3. Mix cooked quinoa with black beans, corn, diced tomatoes, cumin, chili powder, salt, and pepper.

4. Stuff the peppers with the quinoa mixture, top with cheese if desired, and bake for 25-30 minutes until peppers are tender.

Brown Rice Stir-Fry

Ingredients:

- 2 cups cooked brown rice

- 1 cup diced tofu or cooked chicken (if preferred)

- Assorted vegetables (bell peppers, broccoli, carrots, etc.)

- 2 tablespoons gluten-free soy sauce (tamari)

- 1 tablespoon sesame oil

- Minced garlic and ginger

- Green onions for garnish

Nutritional Information (per serving):

Calories	Protein	Carbs	Fat	Fiber
300	12g	40g	10g	8g

Preparation:

1. Heat sesame oil in a pan, sauté garlic and ginger.

2. Add tofu or chicken, cook until lightly browned.

3. Add assorted vegetables, stir-fry until tender-crisp.

4. Mix in cooked brown rice and soy sauce, toss until heated through.

5. Garnish with chopped green onions before serving.

Gluten-Free Spaghetti with Meatballs

Ingredients:

- Gluten-free spaghetti
- Ground beef or turkey
- Gluten-free breadcrumbs
- Egg
- Minced garlic
- Chopped parsley
- Tomato sauce

Nutritional Information (per serving):

Calories	Protein	Carbs	Fat	Fiber
380	20g	40g	15g	6g

Preparation:

1. Cook spaghetti according to package instructions.

2. Mix ground meat with breadcrumbs, egg, garlic, and parsley. Form into meatballs and bake until cooked through.

3. Heat tomato sauce in a pan, add meatballs, and simmer until heated.

4. Serve over cooked spaghetti.

Zucchini Noodles (Zoodles) with Pesto

Ingredients:

- Zucchini, spiralized into noodles
- Homemade or store-bought pesto sauce
- Cherry tomatoes, halved
- Pine nuts
- Grated parmesan cheese (optional)
- Olive oil

Nutritional Information (per serving):

Calories	Protein	Carbs	Fat	Fiber
220	5g	10g	18g	3g

Preparation:

1. In a pan, sauté zucchini noodles with a bit of olive oil until tender.

2. Toss the zoodles with pesto, cherry tomatoes, and pine nuts.

3. Top with grated parmesan if desired before serving.

Chicken and Vegetable Pad Thai

Ingredients:

- Gluten-free rice noodles
- Chicken breast, sliced
- Assorted vegetables (bell peppers, bean sprouts, carrots)
- Pad Thai sauce (gluten-free)
- Lime wedges
- Chopped peanuts

- Chopped cilantro

Nutritional Information (per serving):

Calories	Protein	Carbs	Fat	Fiber
340	25g	45g	8g	5g

Preparation:

1. Cook rice noodles according to package instructions, then drain and set aside.
2. Stir-fry chicken and assorted vegetables until cooked.
3. Add the cooked noodles, Pad Thai sauce, and toss to combine.
4. Serve with lime wedges, chopped peanuts, and cilantro.

Mushroom and Spinach Risotto

Ingredients:

- Arborio rice
- Vegetable broth

- Olive oil

- Chopped onion

- Sliced mushrooms

- Fresh spinach

- Grated parmesan cheese (optional)

- Chopped parsley

Nutritional Information (per serving):

Calories	Protein	Carbs	Fat	Fiber
320	8g	50g	10g	5g

Preparation:

1. In a pot, heat olive oil and sauté onions until translucent.

2. Add mushrooms and cook until softened, then stir in Arborio rice.

3. Gradually add vegetable broth, stirring frequently until rice is cooked and creamy.

4. Stir in fresh spinach and optional parmesan, garnish with parsley before serving.

Lentil and Vegetable Curry with Quinoa

Ingredients:

- Cooked quinoa
- Cooked lentils
- Assorted vegetables (bell peppers, cauliflower, peas)
- Curry sauce (gluten-free)
- Coconut milk
- Olive oil
- Fresh cilantro for garnish

Nutritional Information (per serving):

Calories	Protein	Carbs	Fat	Fiber
340	15g	45g	10g	10g

Preparation:

1. Sauté assorted vegetables in olive oil until tender.

2. Add cooked lentils, curry sauce, and coconut milk, simmer until heated through.

3. Serve over cooked quinoa, garnish with fresh cilantro.

Shrimp and Broccoli Quinoa Stir-Fry

Ingredients:

- Cooked quinoa
- Shrimp, peeled and deveined
- Broccoli florets
- Minced garlic
- Gluten-free soy sauce (tamari)
- Sesame oil
- Red pepper flakes
- Chopped green onions

Nutritional Information (per serving):

Calories	Protein	Carbs	Fat	Fiber
290	25g	30g	8g	6g

Preparation:

1. Sauté shrimp and broccoli in sesame oil with minced garlic until shrimp is pink and broccoli is tender.
2. Add cooked quinoa, soy sauce, and red pepper flakes, toss until heated through.
3. Garnish with chopped green onions before serving.

Hearty Meat and Poultry

Grilled Lemon Herb Chicken

Ingredients:

- Chicken breasts or thighs
- Lemon juice
- Olive oil
- Minced garlic
- Fresh herbs (rosemary, thyme)

- Salt and pepper

Nutritional Information (per serving):

Calories	Protein	Carbs	Fat	Fiber
250	30g	1g	13g	0g

Preparation:

1. In a bowl, mix lemon juice, olive oil, minced garlic, chopped herbs, salt, and pepper.
2. Marinate chicken in the mixture for at least 30 minutes.
3. Grill the chicken until cooked through, basting with the remaining marinade.

Beef Stir-Fry

Ingredients:

- Beef strips (flank or sirloin)
- Assorted vegetables (bell peppers, snap peas, carrots)

- Gluten-free soy sauce (tamari)

- Sesame oil

- Minced ginger and garlic

- Cornstarch (or alternative thickener)

- Green onions for garnish

Nutritional Information (per serving):

Calories	Protein	Carbs	Fat	Fiber
300	25g	15g	15g	5g

Preparation:

1. Toss beef strips with cornstarch, set aside.

2. Stir-fry vegetables in sesame oil, then set aside.

3. In the same pan, cook beef with ginger and garlic until browned.

4. Add vegetables back to the pan, stir in soy sauce, and cook until heated through.

5. Garnish with chopped green onions before serving.

Herb-Crusted Baked Salmon

Ingredients:

- Salmon fillets
- Gluten-free breadcrumbs
- Chopped fresh dill and parsley
- Dijon mustard
- Olive oil
- Lemon wedges

Nutritional Information (per serving):

Calories	Protein	Carbs	Fat	Fiber
280	25g	5g	16g	1g

Preparation:

1. Preheat the oven to 400°F (200°C).
2. Mix breadcrumbs, chopped herbs, and a bit of olive oil to form a paste.

3. Spread mustard on the top of salmon, then press the herb mixture onto the mustard.

4. Bake for 12-15 minutes or until the salmon flakes easily. Serve with lemon wedges.

Pork Tenderloin with Balsamic Glaze

Ingredients:

- Pork tenderloin
- Balsamic vinegar
- Honey
- Minced garlic
- Olive oil
- Salt and pepper

Nutritional Information (per serving):

Calories	Protein	Carbs	Fat	Fiber
270	30g	10g	10g	0g

Preparation:

1. Preheat oven to 375°F (190°C).

2. Season pork with salt and pepper.

3. Sear the pork in a hot pan with olive oil.

4. Transfer to the oven and roast for 20-25 minutes.

5. In a saucepan, simmer balsamic vinegar, honey, and garlic until thickened. Drizzle over the cooked pork.

Roast Turkey Breast

Ingredients:

- Turkey breast
- Garlic powder
- Onion powder
- Paprika
- Olive oil
- Fresh rosemary and thyme
- Salt and pepper

Nutritional Information (per serving):

Calories	Protein	Carbs	Fat	Fiber
230	40g	0g	7g	0g

Preparation:

1. Preheat oven to 350°F (175°C).

2. Rub turkey breast with olive oil, garlic powder, onion powder, paprika, salt, and pepper.

3. Place fresh herbs on and around the turkey.

4. Roast until internal temperature reaches 165°F (74°C).

Glazed Honey Garlic Chicken Thighs

Ingredients:

- Chicken thighs
- Honey
- Gluten-free soy sauce (tamari)
- Minced garlic
- Olive oil

- Sesame seeds for garnish

Nutritional Information (per serving):

Calories	Protein	Carbs	Fat	Fiber
290	25g	15g	15g	0g

Preparation:

1. Mix honey, soy sauce, and minced garlic in a bowl.
2. Coat chicken thighs with the mixture.
3. Heat olive oil in a pan and cook chicken until golden and cooked through.
4. Sprinkle with sesame seeds before serving.

Baked Herb-Crusted Chicken Drumsticks

Ingredients:

- Chicken drumsticks
- Gluten-free breadcrumbs

- Chopped fresh parsley and thyme

- Paprika

- Olive oil

- Salt and pepper

Nutritional Information (per serving):

Calories	Protein	Carbs	Fat	Fiber
240	25g	5g	12g	1g

Preparation:

1. Preheat oven to 400°F (200°C).

2. Mix breadcrumbs, chopped herbs, paprika, olive oil, salt, and pepper in a bowl.

3. Coat drumsticks with the breadcrumb mixture.

4. Bake for 30-35 minutes or until chicken is golden and cooked through.

Lemon Garlic Grilled Shrimp

Ingredients:

- Shrimp, peeled and deveined
- Lemon zest and juice
- Minced garlic
- Olive oil
- Chopped fresh parsley
- Salt and pepper

Nutritional Information (per serving):

Calories	Protein	Carbs	Fat	Fiber
200	20g	2g	12g	0g

Preparation:

1. In a bowl, mix lemon zest, lemon juice, minced garlic, olive oil, chopped parsley, salt, and pepper.
2. Marinate shrimp in the mixture for 15-20 minutes.

3. Grill shrimp over medium heat for 2-3 minutes per side until cooked.

Fish and Seafood Delicacies

Baked Lemon Herb Cod

Ingredients:

- Cod filets
- Lemon juice and zest
- Minced garlic
- Chopped fresh parsley
- Olive oil
- Salt and pepper

Nutritional Information (per serving):

Calories	Protein	Carbs	Fat	Fiber
200	25g	1g	10g	0g

Preparation:

1. Preheat the oven to 400°F (200°C).

2. Mix lemon zest, lemon juice, minced garlic, chopped parsley, olive oil, salt, and pepper in a bowl.

3. Marinate cod filets in the mixture for 15-20 minutes.

4. Place the filets on a baking dish and bake for 15-20 minutes or until the fish flakes easily.

Grilled Salmon with Dill Sauce

Ingredients:

- Salmon fillets
- Dill sauce (mayonnaise, chopped dill, lemon juice)
- Olive oil
- Salt and pepper

Nutritional Information (per serving):

Calories	Protein	Carbs	Fat	Fiber
280	30g	2g	15g	0g

Preparation:

1. Preheat the grill to medium-high heat.

2. Brush salmon with olive oil, season with salt and pepper.

3. Grill salmon for 4-5 minutes on each side or until desired doneness.

4. Serve with dill sauce on the side.

Seared Tuna Steaks

Ingredients:

- Tuna steaks
- Gluten-free soy sauce (tamari)
- Sesame oil
- Minced ginger
- Black and white sesame seeds
- Olive oil
- Salt and pepper

Nutritional Information (per serving):

Calories	Protein	Carbs	Fat	Fiber
250	35g	3g	10g	1g

Preparation:

1. Mix soy sauce, sesame oil, minced ginger, and sesame seeds in a bowl.
2. Marinate tuna steaks in the mixture for 10-15 minutes.
3. Heat olive oil in a pan over high heat and sear tuna for 1-2 minutes per side.
4. Season with salt and pepper before serving.

Pan-Fried Lemon Garlic Halibut

Ingredients:

- Halibut fillets
- Lemon juice and zest
- Minced garlic
- Gluten-free flour (rice flour or alternative)

- Olive oil

- Chopped fresh chives

- Salt and pepper

Nutritional Information (per serving):

Calories	Protein	Carbs	Fat	Fiber
220	30g	5g	8g	1g

Preparation:

1. Season halibut with salt, pepper, lemon zest, and minced garlic.

2. Lightly coat the fish with gluten-free flour.

3. Heat olive oil in a pan over medium heat, then fry halibut for 3-4 minutes per side.

4. Drizzle with lemon juice and garnish with fresh chives before serving.

Shrimp Scampi

Ingredients:

- Shrimp, peeled and deveined

- Minced garlic

- White wine (or chicken broth)

- Lemon juice

- Gluten-free pasta or zoodles

- Butter or olive oil

- Chopped parsley

- Red pepper flakes (optional)

Nutritional Information (per serving):

Calories	Protein	Carbs	Fat	Fiber
280	25g	20g	10g	2g

Preparation:

1. Cook pasta or zoodles according to package instructions, then set aside.

2. In a pan, melt butter or heat olive oil and sauté minced garlic until fragrant.

3. Add shrimp and cook until pink, then remove from the pan.

4. Deglaze the pan with white wine or broth, add lemon juice, and reduce slightly.

5. Toss cooked pasta or zoodles with the shrimp, sauce, and chopped parsley. Add red pepper flakes if desired.

Grilled Lemon Garlic Scallops

Ingredients:

- Scallops
- Lemon juice and zest
- Minced garlic
- Olive oil
- Chopped fresh thyme
- Salt and pepper

Nutritional Information (per serving):

Calories	Protein	Carbs	Fat	Fiber
190	20g	3g	10g	0g

Preparation:

1. In a bowl, mix lemon zest, lemon juice, minced garlic, olive oil, chopped thyme, salt, and pepper.

2. Marinate scallops in the mixture for 10-15 minutes.

3. Preheat the grill to medium-high heat and grill scallops for 2-3 minutes on each side or until opaque.

Lemon Butter Baked Lobster Tails

Ingredients:

- Lobster tails
- Butter, melted
- Lemon juice
- Minced garlic
- Paprika
- Chopped fresh parsley

Nutritional Information (per serving):

Calories	Protein	Carbs	Fat	Fiber
220	25g	2g	12g	0g

Preparation:

1. Preheat oven to 425°F (220°C).

2. Split lobster tails, place them on a baking sheet.

3. Mix melted butter, lemon juice, minced garlic, and paprika. Brush mixture onto the lobster.

4. Bake for 12-15 minutes or until lobster is opaque. Sprinkle with chopped parsley before serving.

Coconut Curry Shrimp

Ingredients:

- Shrimp, peeled and deveined
- Coconut milk
- Red curry paste
- Minced ginger and garlic

- Assorted vegetables (bell peppers, peas, carrots)
- Olive oil
- Chopped cilantro

Nutritional Information (per serving):

Calories	Protein	Carbs	Fat	Fiber
250	20g	10g	15g	3g

Preparation:

1. In a pan, heat olive oil and sauté minced ginger and garlic.
2. Add red curry paste and coconut milk, bring to a simmer.
3. Add assorted vegetables and cook until tender.
4. Stir in shrimp and cook until pink and cooked through. Garnish with chopped cilantro before serving.

CHAPTER 7:

DELICIOUS SIDES

Quinoa and Vegetable Salad

Ingredients:

- Cooked quinoa
- Cherry tomatoes, halved
- Cucumber, diced
- Red onion, finely chopped
- Chopped fresh parsley
- Olive oil and lemon juice for dressing

Nutritional Information (per serving):

Calories	Protein	Carbs	Fat	Fiber
180	5g	30g	6g	5g

Preparation:

1. Combine cooked quinoa, cherry tomatoes, cucumber, red onion, and parsley in a bowl.

2. Drizzle with olive oil and lemon juice, toss well before serving.

Roasted Vegetables

Ingredients:

- Assorted vegetables (bell peppers, zucchini, carrots, etc.)
- Olive oil
- Garlic powder, paprika, salt, and pepper

Nutritional Information (per serving):

Calories	Protein	Carbs	Fat	Fiber
120	3g	15g	7g	5g

Preparation:

1. Preheat oven to 400°F (200°C).

2. Cut vegetables into equal-sized pieces, toss with olive oil, and seasonings.

3. Roast for 25-30 minutes until tender and slightly browned.

Mashed Cauliflower

Ingredients:

- Cauliflower, cut into florets
- Garlic cloves
- Butter or olive oil
- Almond milk (or milk of choice)
- Salt and pepper

Nutritional Information (per serving):

Calories	Protein	Carbs	Fat	Fiber
80	3g	6g	5g	3g

Preparation:

1. Steam or boil cauliflower and garlic until very tender.

2. Mash with butter or olive oil, almond milk, salt, and pepper until desired consistency.

Garlic Herb Quinoa

Ingredients:

- Cooked quinoa
- Minced garlic
- Chopped fresh herbs (parsley, thyme, rosemary)
- Olive oil
- Lemon zest
- Salt and pepper

Nutritional Information (per serving):

Calories	Protein	Carbs	Fat	Fiber
160	5g	25g	5g	3g

Preparation:

1. In a pan, sauté minced garlic with olive
   oil until fragrant.

2. Add cooked quinoa, chopped herbs,
   lemon zest, salt, and pepper. Mix well
   and serve.

Sautéed Spinach with Pine Nuts

Ingredients:

- Fresh spinach leaves
- Pine nuts
- Olive oil
- Minced garlic
- Salt and pepper

Nutritional Information (per serving):

Calories	Protein	Carbs	Fat	Fiber
90	4g	3g	7g	2g

Preparation:

1. Toast pine nuts in a pan until golden, then set aside.

2. Sauté minced garlic in olive oil until aromatic.

3. Add spinach and cook until wilted. Season with salt and pepper.

4. Sprinkle with toasted pine nuts before serving.

Glazed Carrots

Ingredients:

- Carrots, peeled and sliced
- Maple syrup or honey
- Butter or dairy-free alternative
- Chopped parsley (optional)

Nutritional Information (per serving):

Calories	Protein	Carbs	Fat	Fiber
100	1g	15g	5g	3g

Preparation:

1. Boil or steam carrots until tender, then drain.

2. In a pan, melt butter, add maple syrup or honey, and cooked carrots.

3. Cook until the glaze thickens and coats the carrots. Garnish with parsley if desired.

Cucumber Tomato Salad

Ingredients:

- Cucumbers, sliced
- Cherry tomatoes, halved
- Red onion, thinly sliced
- Chopped fresh dill
- Olive oil and red wine vinegar for dressing
- Salt and pepper

Nutritional Information (per serving):

Calories	Protein	Carbs	Fat	Fiber
70	2g	8g	4g	2g

Preparation:

1. Combine cucumbers, tomatoes, onion, and dill in a bowl.
2. Drizzle with olive oil, red wine vinegar, salt, and pepper. Toss well before serving.

Steamed Asparagus with Lemon Butter

Ingredients:

- Asparagus spears
- Butter or dairy-free alternative
- Lemon juice and zest
- Salt and pepper

Nutritional Information (per serving):

Calories	Protein	Carbs	Fat	Fiber

60	4g	5g	4g	3g

Preparation:

1. Steam asparagus until tender-crisp, then set aside.
2. In a pan, melt butter, add lemon zest, lemon juice, salt, and pepper.
3. Drizzle over the steamed asparagus before serving.

Oven-Roasted Brussels Sprouts

Ingredients:

- Brussels sprouts, halved
- Olive oil
- Balsamic vinegar
- Minced garlic
- Salt and pepper

Nutritional Information (per serving):

Calories	Protein	Carbs	Fat	Fiber

90	4g	12g	4g	4g

Preparation:

1. Toss Brussels sprouts with olive oil, balsamic vinegar, minced garlic, salt, and pepper.
2. Roast in the oven at 400°F (200°C) for 20-25 minutes until caramelized and crispy.

Herbed Rice Pilaf

Ingredients:

- Cooked white or brown rice
- Chopped almonds or pine nuts
- Chopped fresh herbs (parsley, dill, thyme)
- Olive oil
- Lemon juice
- Salt and pepper

Nutritional Information (per serving):

Calories	Protein	Carbs	Fat	Fiber
150	3g	20g	6g	2g

Preparation:

1. In a pan, toast nuts in olive oil until golden, then set aside.
2. Add cooked rice, chopped herbs, lemon juice, salt, and pepper. Stir well and top with the toasted nuts before serving.

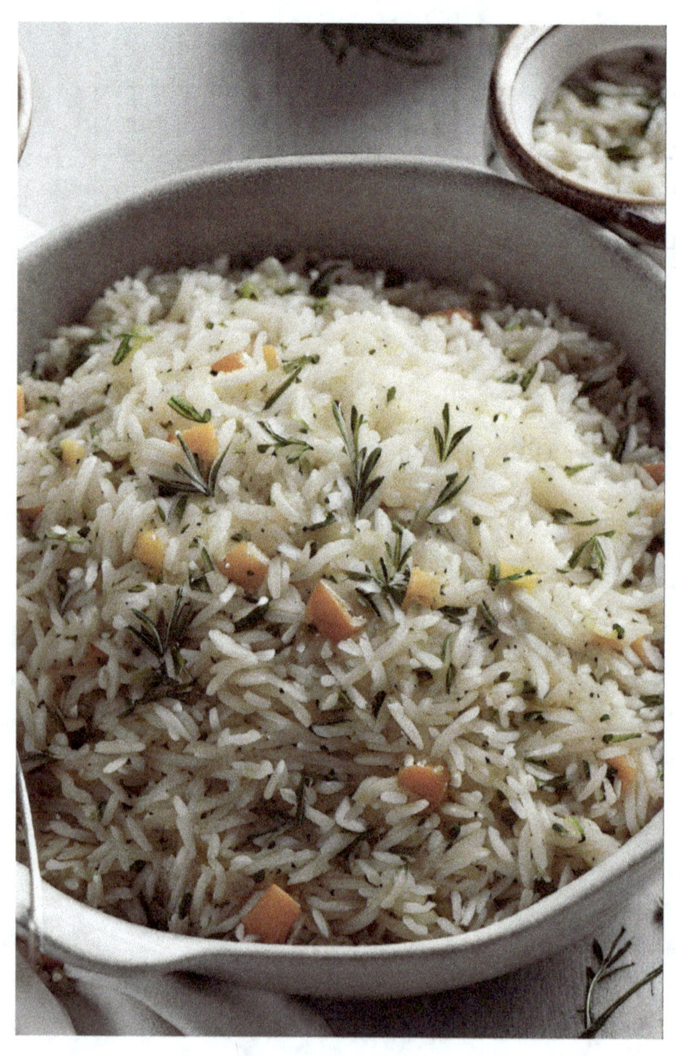

CHAPTER 8:

SWEET TREATS AND DESSERTS

Flourless Chocolate Cake

Ingredients:

- Dark chocolate (70% cocoa or higher)
- Butter or dairy-free alternative
- Eggs
- Sugar or sweetener of choice
- Cocoa powder
- Vanilla extract

Nutritional Information (per serving):

Calories	Protein	Carbs	Fat	Fiber
250	5g	20g	18g	3g

Preparation:

1. Preheat the oven to 350°F (175°C) and grease a cake pan.

2. Melt chocolate and butter together in a bowl.

3. In another bowl, beat eggs and sugar until fluffy, then add cocoa powder and vanilla extract.

4. Combine the two mixtures, pour into the cake pan, and bake for 25-30 minutes.

Fruit Parfait

Ingredients:

- Greek yogurt or dairy-free yogurt
- Mixed fruits (berries, chopped mango, kiwi, etc.)
- Gluten-free granola
- Honey or maple syrup (optional)

Nutritional Information (per serving):

Calories	Protein	Carbs	Fat	Fiber

Calories	Protein	Carbs	Fat	Fiber
180	8g	30g	4g	5g

Preparation:

1. Layer yogurt, mixed fruits, and granola in a glass or bowl.
2. Drizzle with honey or maple syrup for added sweetness if desired.

Coconut Macaroons

Ingredients:

- Shredded coconut
- Sweetened condensed milk (check for gluten-free)
- Egg whites
- Vanilla extract
- Salt

Nutritional Information (per serving):

Calories	Protein	Carbs	Fat	Fiber

120	2g	10g	8g	1g

Preparation:

1. Preheat oven to 325°F (160°C) and line a baking sheet with parchment paper.

2. Mix shredded coconut, condensed milk, egg whites, vanilla extract, and salt in a bowl.

3. Scoop spoonfuls onto the baking sheet and bake for 20-25 minutes or until golden.

Almond Flour Chocolate Chip Cookies

Ingredients:

- Almond flour
- Baking soda
- Salt
- Butter or coconut oil
- Brown sugar or coconut sugar
- Eggs

- Vanilla extract

- Chocolate chips (check for gluten-free)

Nutritional Information (per serving - 2 cookies):

Calories	Protein	Carbs	Fat	Fiber
160	3g	15g	10g	2g

Preparation:

1. Preheat the oven to 350°F (175°C) and line a baking sheet with parchment paper.
2. Mix almond flour, baking soda, and salt in a bowl.
3. In another bowl, cream butter and sugar, then add eggs and vanilla.
4. Combine both mixtures, add chocolate chips, and spoon onto the baking sheet. Bake for 10-12 minutes.

Rice Pudding

Ingredients:

- Cooked white rice
- Milk or almond milk
- Sugar or sweetener of choice
- Cinnamon
- Raisins (optional)
- Vanilla extract

Nutritional Information (per serving):

Calories	Protein	Carbs	Fat	Fiber
200	4g	35g	4g	1g

Preparation:

1. In a pot, combine rice, milk, sugar, and cinnamon. Simmer until thickened.
2. Stir in raisins and vanilla extract. Serve warm or chilled.

Homemade Berry Sorbet

Ingredients:

- Mixed berries (strawberries, blueberries, raspberries)
- Lemon juice
- Honey or agave syrup

Nutritional Information (per serving):

Calories	Protein	Carbs	Fat	Fiber
100	1g	25g	0.5g	5g

Preparation:

1. Blend mixed berries, lemon juice, and sweetener in a blender until smooth.
2. Pour into a shallow dish and freeze for a few hours, stirring occasionally until set.

Banana Chocolate Popsicles

Ingredients:

- Ripe bananas

- Cocoa powder

- Almond milk or any milk of choice

- Honey or maple syrup

Nutritional Information (per serving):

Calories	Protein	Carbs	Fat	Fiber
90	2g	20g	1g	3g

Preparation:

1. Blend bananas, cocoa powder, milk, and sweetener until smooth.

2. Pour into popsicle molds and freeze until solid.

Frozen Yogurt Bark

Ingredients:

- Greek yogurt or dairy-free yogurt

- Honey or agave syrup

- Fresh fruits, nuts, shredded coconut

Nutritional Information (per serving):

Calories	Protein	Carbs	Fat	Fiber
120	6g	15g	4g	2g

Preparation:

1. Mix yogurt and sweetener, spread onto a baking sheet lined with parchment paper.

2. Sprinkle with chopped fruits, nuts, or shredded coconut. Freeze until firm, then break into pieces.

Pumpkin Spice Muffins

Ingredients:

- Gluten-free flour blend
- Baking powder
- Pumpkin puree
- Brown sugar or coconut sugar
- Eggs
- Pumpkin pie spice
- Vanilla extract

Nutritional Information (per serving):

Calories	Protein	Carbs	Fat	Fiber
150	3g	25g	5g	2g

Preparation:

1. Preheat the oven to 350°F (175°C) and line a muffin tin with paper liners.

2. Mix flour, baking powder, pumpkin puree, sugar, eggs, pumpkin pie spice, and vanilla.

3. Fill muffin cups and bake for 20-25 minutes.

CHAPTER 9:

EMBRACING A GLUTEN-FREE LIFESTYLE

Before You Go:

1. **Research Ahead:** Check the restaurant's website or call ahead to understand their gluten-free options. Many restaurants now provide specific gluten-free menus or label items that are safe for consumption.

2. **Ask Around:** Utilize resources like social media or local community groups to ask for recommendations from others who follow a gluten-free diet. They might suggest restaurants with great options.

At The Restaurant:

1. **Communication is Key:** When you arrive, communicate your dietary needs clearly to the server. Explain your gluten-free requirements, emphasizing the severity of your intolerance or allergy.

2. **Understand The Menu:** Review the menu thoroughly, looking for dishes that are naturally gluten-free or can be easily modified. Grilled meats, fish, vegetables, and salads are often safer options.

3. **Question Ingredients and Preparation:** Ask about specific ingredients, cooking methods, and any potential cross-contamination risks. Inquire about marinades, sauces, and whether items are cooked in shared fryers or on shared surfaces.

4. **Be Cautious of Cross-Contamination:** Be aware of potential cross-

contamination risks in the kitchen. Even if a dish seems gluten-free, it might have come into contact with gluten during preparation.

5. **Substitute Wisely:** If a dish comes with a gluten-containing side, inquire about swapping it for a safe alternative. For instance, ask for a salad instead of bread or opt for steamed vegetables instead of pasta.

Etiquette and Precautions:

1. **Be Patient and Kind:** Some restaurant staff might not be fully informed about gluten-free requirements. Be patient and understanding, but firm about your dietary needs.

2. **Don't Hesitate to Ask:** If you're uncertain about any dish, don't hesitate to ask for clarification. It's crucial to have confidence in what you're consuming.

3. **Double-Check Before Eating:** Even if you've ordered a gluten-free meal, double-check the dish when it arrives to ensure it aligns with your needs.

Takeaways:

1. **Trust Your Gut:** If you feel unsure about a restaurant's ability to accommodate your gluten-free needs, it might be better to opt for another dining establishment where you feel more confident.

2. **Enjoy the Experience:** Despite the precautions, dining out should be an enjoyable experience. Focus on the company, the ambiance, and the joy of exploring different culinary experiences while keeping your health a priority.

Managing Social Situations

Potlucks Or Gatherings:

1. **Communicate in Advance:** If attending a potluck or gathering, let the host know about your gluten-free dietary needs. Offer to bring a dish that you can enjoy and share with others.

2. **Prepare a Dish:** Consider preparing a gluten-free dish that you'll enjoy and that others can try. This way, you're certain of having at least one safe option.

3. **Choose Safe Options:** When faced with the offerings at the event, opt for dishes that are most likely to be gluten-free, such as salads, fruits, vegetables, and non-breaded proteins.

Dining Out with Friends or Family:

1. **Suggest Safe Restaurants:** When making plans to dine out, suggest restaurants known for their gluten-free

options or flexibility in accommodating dietary needs. Check menus in advance.

2. **Explain Your Needs:** Inform your friends or family about your dietary requirements beforehand. Discuss your concerns and share information about gluten intolerance to ensure understanding and support.

3. **Guide Restaurant Selection:** Offer to help select the restaurant or suggest a few options that cater well to gluten-free diets. Look for places with clearly labeled gluten-free choices.

Social Events and Parties:

1. **BYO Snacks:** If you're uncertain about available options at a social event or party, bring your own snacks or small meal to ensure you have something safe to eat.

2. **Talk to the Host:** Politely talk to the host about your dietary needs. They might be willing to accommodate or let you know in advance about any safe options available.

3. **Eat Beforehand:** If attending a social event where gluten-free options might be limited, have a meal or snack beforehand so you aren't solely reliant on what's available.

Maintaining A Positive Attitude:

1. **Focus on Socializing:** Instead of making food the main focus, concentrate on enjoying the company, conversations, and activities at social events.

2. **Be Confident in Your Needs:** Don't feel pressured to consume something you're uncertain about. Your health is a priority, and it's okay to politely decline if

something doesn't align with your dietary requirements.

3. **Educate and Advocate:** Use these opportunities to educate others about gluten intolerance and the challenges of maintaining a gluten-free diet. It can foster understanding and support from those around you.

Staying Healthy and Happy

Nutrition:

1. **Balanced Diet:** Ensure your gluten-free diet is well-rounded with a variety of fruits, vegetables, lean proteins, and gluten-free whole grains to meet your nutritional needs.

2. **Reading Labels:** Familiarize yourself with reading food labels to identify gluten-containing ingredients and hidden

sources of gluten, ensuring your choices are safe.

3. **Gluten-Free Substitutes:** Experiment with gluten-free alternatives for your favorite foods. Try quinoa, brown rice, almond flour, and other gluten-free options to diversify your meals.

Emotional Health:

1. **Stay Positive:** Embrace your gluten-free lifestyle positively, focusing on the delicious and nutritious options available rather than feeling restricted.

2. **Seek Support:** Join support groups, online communities, or forums where you can connect with others who follow a gluten-free diet. Share experiences, tips, and recipes.

3. **Manage Stress:** Incorporate stress-reducing practices like meditation, yoga, or deep breathing to manage stress, which can impact your overall health.

Lifestyle:

1. **Regular Exercise:** Engage in regular physical activity that you enjoy. It not only contributes to good health but also aids in stress reduction and overall well-being.

2. **Adequate Sleep:** Prioritize sleep for overall health. Good sleep patterns help manage stress and support a strong immune system.

3. **Hydration:** Drink plenty of water throughout the day to support overall health and proper bodily functions.

Self-Care:

1. **Celebrate Small Victories:** Acknowledge and celebrate your achievements in maintaining a gluten-free lifestyle. Small wins add up to a healthier, happier you.

2. **Treat Yourself:** Find ways to indulge in gluten-free treats and desserts that you enjoy. Having a favorite gluten-free treat can boost your happiness.

3. **Consult a Professional:** If needed, consult a registered dietitian or healthcare professional specializing in gluten-free diets for guidance and support.

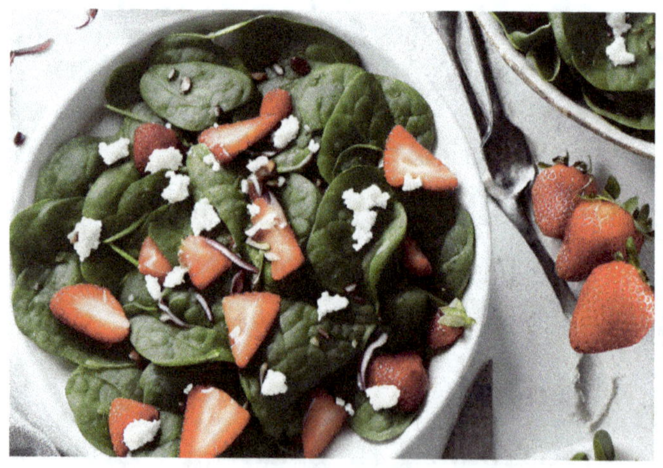

Your experience matters! If you've found value in the recipes and insights provided in the 'CELIAC DISEASE COOKBOOK,' I invite you to share your thoughts and feelings about the book. Your review not only helps others discover a resource that could significantly impact their lives but also supports our shared journey toward a healthier, gluten-free lifestyle. Your feedback is invaluable and will inspire others to explore this essential guide. Your honest review will guide and encourage fellow celiac sufferers on their path to wellness. Thank you for taking the time to share your thoughts and for being part of this community dedicated to embracing a fulfilling, gluten-free life.

www.ingramcontent.com/pod-product-compliance
Lightning Source LLC
Chambersburg PA
CBHW070949260726
48661CB00003B/1197